The Complete Ketogenic Diet Cookbook for Beginners

70 Budget-Friendly Ketogenic (Keto) Recipes

30-Day Diet Meal Plan

ISBN- **978-1981971640**
ISBN- **1981971645**

Dedication

This book is dedicated to those who are willing to help themselves. I also dedicate this book to my family and friends.

Table of Contents

Breakfast 28

Quick scrambled eggs 28

Scrambled eggs with guacamole 30

Asparagus and egg 31

Salad with chicken breast and spinach 32

Bacon lemon thyme breakfast muffins 33

Cheese omelet with bacon 34

Fried eggs with cheese and nuts 36

Protein pancakes with cottage cheese 37

Snacks 38

Spicy egg sandwich 38

Chicken burrito 39

Stuffed eggs 40

Broccoli with Tofu 42

Pepper stuffed with cottage cheese 43

Meat rolls without cooking 44

Soft Tacos with Chicken and Avocado 45

Taco with fried cod and salsa 46

Lunch 47

Tamari marinated steak salad 47

Bacon wrapped chicken with garlic 48

Easy zucchini beef sauté with garlic and coriander 50

Soups & Stews 52

Chicken Noodle Soup 52

Broccoli & curry cream soup 53

Soup with Poached Egg 54

Beef stew with mushrooms and vegetables 55

Mushroom cream soup 57

Cabbage & zucchini soup 58

Chicken Soup with bacon and mushrooms 60

Stewed chicken livers 61

Cream soup with shrimp 62

Dinner 63

Cauliflower taboule salad 63

Beef curry 64

Thai Chicken with cauliflower rice 66

Grilled chicken skewers with garlic sauce 69

Pasta with chicken and basil 71

Meat 72

Pork steak with parmesan 72

Meat rolls 73

Pan-fried pork tenderloin 74

Chicken with pesto and cream cheese 75

Fish & Seafood 77

Baked salmon with orange juice 77

Fried cod 78

Tuna salad 79

Mustard sardine salad 80

Baked tilapia fillet 82

Veggies 83

Broccoli Salad 83

Spinach stir-fry 84

Stuffed zucchini 85

Mushroom casserole 86

Introduction

Many people who control their weight may notice that refraining from flour, sweets, potatoes and cereals helps to lose several extra pounds. That is because of rapid restriction of carbohydrates. Not having received the daily portion of glucose that you are used to having, your body begins to look for other sources of energy and finally settles on fats and proteins.

Several years ago, lots of people were crazy about the low-carbohydrate diets. Later those were discredited. It seems that the pendulum stopped swinging: the nutritionists concluded that the optimal, and safest weight loss regimen is a **ketogenic diet**. In addition to the sensational Kremlin's and Atkins'diets, it is stricter, but at the same time more effective. The Keto diet recently became one of the most popular, one of the most mystic and most discussed diets, as it gives the best results in shorter terms.

Modern society looses weight actively by eating homemade mayonnaise, and even by ordering keto burgers which look like the tastiest burger one could ever have.

More than 20 researchers according to Authority Nutrition, proved the benefit of that diet for losing weight and for good health as well. It is also used as a method of treatment for cancer, diabetes, epilepsy and Alzheimer's disease.

The top figure in the popularization of these scientific results and the brilliant interpreter, is a science writer and a reviewer, Garry Taubes. Gradually he proved that people put on weight, not because of eating a lot, but started eating a lot because of putting on weight. How weird is that? He saw the only one way out of that trap to be insulin jumps.

This book is a guide about the keto diet, not just a cookbook. All recipes are easy to prepare. Ingredients are simple — you can find them in every store. Different kinds of spices are esay to find and affordable. You can also combine or substitute some ingredients. You will find a variety of simple recipes. The preparation time, cooking time, and calory count of each dish is indicated

Carbohydrates increase the amount of sugar in our blood. Our body converts most of them into the sugar glucose, which is absorbed into the bloodstream.

There are two forms of carbohydrates: sugars (such as fructose, glucose, and lactose) and starches, which are found in foods such as starchy vegetables (potatoes), grains, rice, bread, and cereals.

Insulin is a hormone that moves sugar from the blood into cells, where it is used as a source of energy. It is released by the pancreas.

Proteins are the most important macro. They are essential, and necessary to produce all the amino acids we require. ,And proteins are required for doing most of the work in cells: building and rebuilding all of our soft tissues and organs.

Electrolytes are the medical term for salts or ion which carry an electric charge and are found in the blood and other body fluds.

In biological systems, the electrolytes are: Sodium $(Na+)$, Calcium $(Ca+2)$, Chloride $(Cl-)$.

Magnesium $(Mg+2)$ is used in almost every chemical process in your body. It is found in nuts and seeds (walnuts, almonds, pistachios, sesame, pecans, and pumpkin seeds).

Potassium $(K+)$ is also a major electrolyte that is used in different kinds of muscle contractions and by your organs. Green leafy vegetables and avocados contain it.

Chapter 1

What is a ketogenic diet?

The ketogenic diet (keto diet) was developed in the 1980s. Then bodybuilding was a very popular activity, and used by sportsmen for building muscle.
The ketogenic diet is a very low-carb diet, which burns fats in your body.

How does it work?

The first principle is the restriction of carbohydrates. They are the main souce of energy for our bodies If carbohydrate intake is stopped, the process of getting energy turns to stored fats. That state is called **ketosis**. As a result, weight loss happens, not because of muscle tissues decreasing or excretion of water from it, but due to losing fat.

.

Top 7 keto mistakes

Almost everyone makes mistakes! Here are the most common keto mistakes:

Getting impatient with adaptation

Before you jump into a keto diet, you have to understand that you've been running on carbohydrates your entire life. Now your body has to switch metabolism entirely and start converting fat into energy instead of using carbs. Don't be impatient!

1. Not getting enough electrolytes

Electrolytes are essential, but definitely they're necessary for this diet. If you don't have enough sodium, magnesium, vitamin D, salt and potassium in your diet, you will experience headaches, fatigue, constipation, lethargy — the so-called "keto flu". This may be the number one reason why most people quit the diet. Your body needs plenty of these nutrients while you're on a keto diet.

2. Not meal planning

This may be one of the biggest mistake. Those who do not plan meals end up failing because they are hungry. Sure, it takes time to create the meal plan, but nobody said this was going to be a walk in the park. Meal planning saves you from headaches and frustration, but, also, it's a great way to save your money as well, because you have planned ahead what you are going to buy.

3. Comparing yourself to others

Stop. Just stop. You and I are unique people! Everybody has his or her different relationships with food, diets and eating histories. Someone else's progress is not a determining factor in your success.

Your body reacts differently from someone else. You can reach common outcomes such as weight loss, energy, etc. at different times because of many various factors which affect your results. Just focus on *you*, and what you need to do to succeed.

4. Not drinking enough water

Without water, your body can't do what it's supposed to do. You have to drink more water than you are used to, so, this can be quite challenging for some people. So, how much water should you drink? The general rule is 0.5 oz to 1 oz for every pound of bodyweight per day

5. Not getting enough sleep

Just like water, without sleeping enough, your body can't do what it needs to do. Changing your lifestyle is hard enough!

6. Not willing to bend the rules

Sometimes you can ignore the rules! You have to listen to your body or heart, have to know yourself well enough to know what types of food to eat and when, (of course, you should always check with your doctor for advice). When your best friend or relatives invite you to a restaurant, you don't have to refuse going there just because you are on a diet. Don't be a slave to rules! When you get home, you get right back on plan.

Types of ketogenic diets

There are several variants of the ketogenic diet.

- **Standard keto diet**. It means a low-carbohydrate intake (5%), a moderately level of proteins (20%), and a high intake of fats (75%).
- **Cyclic keto.** This type includes intermittent periods of carbohydrate loading. For example, five days of the keto diet and two days of the normal diet.
- **Purpose keto diet** allows adding carbohydrates during physical training days.
- **High protein keto diet.** That type includes a lot of proteins. The macro ratio: 60% fats, 35% proteins, 5% carbs.

The benefits of keto

- Helps to lose weight;
- You don't have to calculate calories — it will work efficiently anyway;
- Eating a lot of protein keeps you from being hungry;
- Decreases blood sugar levels and increases the response to insulin.

Who should NOT do keto?

- Those who are suffering from diabetes;
- Those who have high blood pressure;

- Pregnant women and breastfeeding mothers;
- Those who have problems with the thyroid gland;
- Those who have problems with kidneys, liver and gastrointestinal problems.

Ketosis: what you have to know about it

Although the keto diet is safe for healthy people, it is not right for everyone. Some might observe several side effects while the body is adapting to the new state of living.

After several days (2-5, sometimes more) of eating low carbs and high fat, you may not feel comfortable. Without carbs, you may be in a bad mood — everything and everybody irritates you. Lethargy, decreased appetite, sickness, and weakness may occur, especially, in autumn. That is why women shouldn't start keto before menstruation, during it, and in a stressful period of life..

"Keto flu" is the first sign of ketosis. That could manifest as a headache, foggy thinking, fatigue, etc. Drink plenty of water and eat plenty of salt.

There is no doubt, for people who are used to eating lots of vegetables, increasing fat consumption may be stressful. Only people who live in northen climes can eat a high-fat diet regularly without damaging their health.

The keto diet is a natural diuretic, and you'll urinate more often than before. Keep on consuming salt and a plenty of water, and allow your body to rehydrate and resupply your electrolytes. Doing this will help you with the headaches or even eliminate them completely.

Constipation also may happen, mostly in the early stages. If it occurs, follow these few suggestions:

- Drink more water and eat more leafy greens and other high-fiber vegetables
- Eat 1-2 tablespoons of coconut oil every day (also helps keep you full).
- Make sure your salt intake is high enough.

Chapter 2

Keto diet food list: what to eat and what to avoid

In the keto diet, the accent is on using fats and avoiding carbohydrates.

Meat/Seafood
Organic chicken breasts/thighs (skin-on has a higher fat content), pepperoni, grass fed 85% lean ground beef, sausages, bacon, turkey, roast beef, salmon, tuna, tilapia, shrimp, crab, lobster, pork, chicken and beef broths, seaweed.

Dairy
Eggs, pasture-raised butter or ghee, full-fat cheeses (cheddar, provolone, mozzarella, parmesan), full-fat cream cheese, full-fat sour cream, heavy cream.

Greens
Leafy greens (spinach, kale, romaine, lettuce, iceberg), bell peppers, cucumbers, jalapeños, zucchini, celery, mushrooms, onions, asparagus, Brussels sprouts, broccoli, green beans, red pepper, cauliflower, garlic, avocados, herbs. Small amounts of raspberries, blackberries, blueberries, strawberries.

Grocery items
Tuna (canned), mayonnaise. Natural peanut butter

with no sugar (if it is possible), olive oil (extra virgin preferably), coconut and avocado oils. Tomato sauce/paste, **tamari soy sauce (gluten-free)**. Almond and coconut flours; baking powder, unsweetened cocoa powder; vanilla or vanilla extract, chia seeds, raw almonds, macadamia nuts, pickles. Stevia (that is the natural sweetener), apple cider vinegar, almond milk, hot sauce., full-fat dressing.

Foods to Avoid
Bread, pasta, quinoa, candy, pizza, ice cream, oats, pre-made sauces, margarine, bakery foods, potatoes, barley, rye, corn, beans, peas, lentils, rice, and other starchy vegetables, most processed food, beer and dessert wine. Develop your creativity: experiment, and you'll fall out of love with bread, pizza, and other comfort foods.

For those who follow the keto diet, fruits are limited because of containing lots of carbs and sugar. Eating sour fruits in little amounts is possible. You can usually consume 1/2 cup of berries without issue, but other fruits are typically off limits.

What to drink

So, what do you drink on keto? Water is perfect, coffee and tea too. Don't use sweeteners. Using a little milk or cream is OK. The occasional glass of wine is possible, **too. Tea can add many health benefits as does coffee.**

Advice for the beginners

Don't be afraid to follow keto if you are a vegetarian. It is quite possible.

The strategy: Divide 1600 calories into three meals, and the three meals into three snacks. You feel satiated all day. Eat every 2-3 hours to avoid hunger. It is necessary to follow a diet plan such as the following: 2.5g protein, 1g fat, 1g carbohydrate per 1 kg body weight per day.

Try to alternate the food every day so that you get more vitamins and macro elements.

NOTE: Keto isn't a doctor. If you have some pre-existing medical conditions which might not work well with a keto plan, please consult a qualified medical professional.

Chapter 3 — Recipes

Smoothies & Breakfast

All the recipes are for one person.
Always try to add new vegetables and meat (fish) to prevent the lack of nutrients. Create your plan according to following recipes.
Some abbreviations used:
Tablespoon – Tbs;
Teaspoon – tsp;
1 cup – 8 oz or 240 ml;
Ounce — oz
Pound — lb

Smoothies

Keto smoothie with avocado

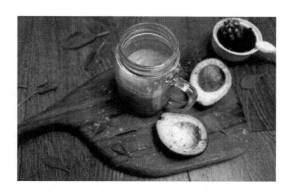

Ingredients:

- 1 avocado;
- 1 banana;
- 1 cup of full-fat cream or kefir;
- 1¾ oz of spinach;
- 1 tsp of matcha;
- 2 Tbs of coconut oil;
- Stevia to taste

How to prepare:

Put all the ingredients in a blender. Pour the smoothie into cups and enjoy!
Preparation time: 5 minutes
Cooking time: 5 minutes
Total time: 10 minutes
Calories: 98 | Fat: 7g | Carbohydrates: 5g | Protein: 1g

Keto Green smoothie

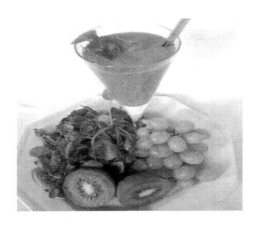

Ingredients:

- 1 kiwi fruit;
- 20 sour grapes;
- 1 carrot;
- 1 oz of spinach;
- fresh coriander leaves.

Kiwi is the best alternative for those who have an allergy to citrus. Grapes are full of vitamins.

How to prepare:

Peel the kiwi and the carrot. Cut them into pieces. Add spinach and fresh coriander leaves. Blend it all. You can serve it with a couple of ice cubes.

Preparation time: 5-7 minutes
Cooking time: 5 minutes
Total time: 10-12 minutes

Keto Green Smoothie with nuts

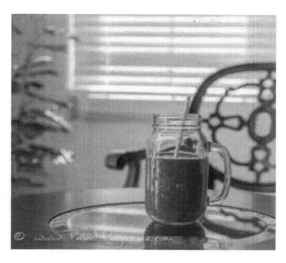

Ingredients:

- 1¾ oz spinach;
- 8 almonds, raw;
- 2 walnuts or brazil nuts;
- 1 cup unsweetened coconut milk

How to prepare:

Put the ingredients into a blender and blend them welll.
Preparation time: 5 minutes
Cooking time: 5 minutes
Total time: 10 minutes
Nutrition Information:
Calories: 380 | Fat: 30g | Carbohydrates: 13g | Sugar: 3g |
Fiber: 8g | Protein: 12g

Smoothie with Matcha

Matcha is a Japanese green tea. Leaves ground into a powder contain plenty of antioxidants, much more than in ordinary green tea.

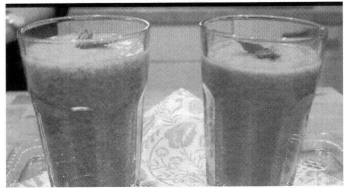

Ingredients:

1 tsp matcha powder;
1 cup coconut yogurt;
½ cup of berries (frozen may be used);
1 Tbs coconut flakes;
1 Tbs cocoa nibs;
Stevia.

How to prepare:

Add the matcha powder to the yogurt. If you prefer a sweet smoothie, you can add Stevia. Blend it. Pour the smoothie into a glass. Top with the berries, coconut flakes, and cocoa nibs.
Preparation time: 5 minutes
Cooking time: 5 minutes
Total time: 10 minutes
Nutrition Information:
Calories: 127 | Fat: 10g | Carbohydrates: 10g | Sugar: 5g | Protein: 3g

Lemon smoothie with banana and strawberries

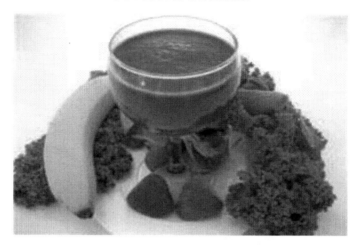

Ingredients:

- 1 banana;
- 5-6 strawberries;
- mint leaves;
- 1 kiwi fruit;
- ¾ oz spinach.

How to prepare:

Wash all the ingredients. Peel the banana and the kiwi. Put all ingredients in a blender and mix.
Preparation time: 5-7 minutes
Cooking time: 5 minutes
Total time: 10-12 minutes
Calories: 68 | Fat: 0 | Carbohydrates: 13g | Fiber: 1g | Protein: 1g

Lime & Pear Smoothie

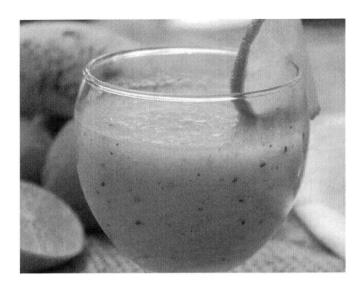

Ingredients:

- 1/2 of a lime;
- 1 pear;
- 1¾ oz spinach;
- 1¾ oz water (or high-fat kefir).

How to prepare:

Wash all the ingredients. Cut the pear into halves and remove the core. Put the ingredients in a blender and blend them together. You can serve in a cup or glass, and add a couple of ice cubes.

Preparation time: 5 minutes
Cooking time: 5 minutes
Total time: 10 minutes
Calories: 25 | Fat: 0.3g | Carbohydrates: 5g | Fiber: 1g | Protein: 0.5g

Smoothie with avocado

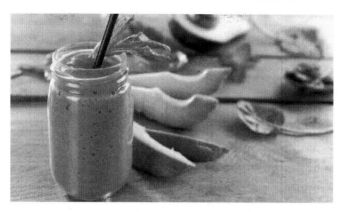

Ingredients:

- 1 ripe avocado;
- 1 middle size cucumber;
- 3 cloves of garlic;
- ½ of lemon;
- 5 stalks of celery
- 5 leaves of fresh coriander;
- salt to taste.

How to prepare:

Wash and then peel the cucumber and the avocado. Put all the ingredients in a blender. Blend them well.
Preparation time: 10 minutes
Cooking time: 5 minutes
Total time: 15 minutes
Calories: 132 | Fat: 11g | Carbohydrates: 5g | Fiber: 1g | Protein: 2g

Breakfast

Quick scrambled eggs

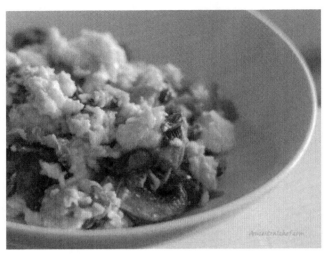

Ingredients:

3 eggs, whisked;
4 baby Bella mushrooms;
¼ cup red bell peppers;
½ cup of spinach;
2 slices of ham;
1 Tbs of coconut oil or ghee;
salt and pepper to taste.

How to prepare:

Chop up the vegetables and the ham. Put ½
Tbs of coconut oil or ghee in a frying pan and
melt. Add all ingredients except the eggs. Sauté

until tender. Put the whisked eggs into a separate frying pan with the other ½ Tbs of coconut oil or ghee. Cook on medium heat while stirring. Once the eggs are cooked, add salt and pepper to taste. Mix everything together. Serve immediately.

Preparation time: 10 minutes
Cooking time: 10 minutes
Total time: 20 minutes

Nutrition Information:

Serving size: 1 plate
Calories: 350 | Fat: 29g | Carbohydrates: 5g | Sugar: 3g | Fiber: 1g | Protein: 21g

Scrambled eggs with guacamole

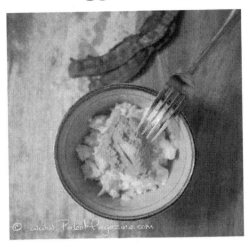

Ingredients:

3 eggs;
1 Tbs of coconut oil;
¼ cup guacamole (you can make it or buy it);
a pinch of salt.

How to prepare:

Heat the oil in a pan. Scramble the eggs over a low heat. Top them with the guacamole. You can add salt to taste.

Preparation time: 5 minutes
Cooking time: 5-10 minutes
Total time: 10-15 minutes
Nutrition Information:
Calories: 370 | Fat: 23g | Carbohydrates: 4g | Sugar: 1g | Fiber: 2g | Protein:18g

Asparagus and egg

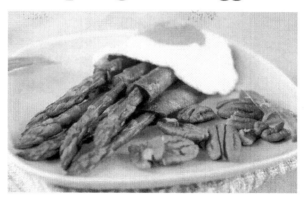

Ingredients:

- 5-6 asparagus shoots;
- 2-3 walnuts;
- 1 egg;
- 5-6 slices of ham;
- 1 Tbs of olive oil;
- salt, pepper, and lemon juice to taste.

How to prepare:

Wash asparagus shoots thoroughly. Cut off the hard ends. Dry them with the kitchen towel. Grease a baking dish with the oil and place asparagus in it. Add salt and pepper. Bake for about 15 minutes. Wrap each asparagus shoot with a slice of ham. Sprinkle with the lemon juice.

Preparation time: 10-15 minutes
Cooking time: 15 minutes
Total time: 25-30 minutes
Calories: 240 | Carbohydrates: 8g | Sugar: 0

Salad with chicken breast and spinach

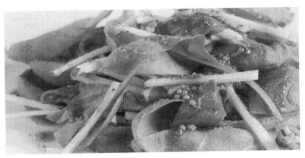

Ingredients:

- 3.5 oz chicken breast;
- 2 Tbs of spinach;
- 1¾ oz of lettuce;
- 1 bell pepper;
- 2 Tbs of olive oil;
- lemon juice to taste

How to prepare:

Boil the chicken breast without adding salt, and then cut it into small strips. Put the spinach in boiling water for a few minutes, then cut it into small strips, also. Cut the pepper in strips as well. Mix all the ingredients, add oil and juice. You can even boil chicken in advance, so that saves your time and shortens the preparation time quite a lot.

Preparation time: 30 minutes
Cooking time: 25 minutes
Total time: 30-55 minutes
Nutrition information:
Calories: 100 | Fat: 11g | Carbohydrates: 3g | Fiber: 2g | Protein: 6g

Bacon lemon thyme breakfast muffins

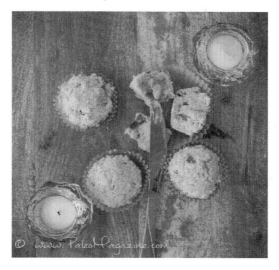

Ingredients:

- 3 cups of almond flour;
- 1 cup bacon cut into pieces.
- ½ cup of ghee, melted;
- 4 eggs;
- 2 tsp lemon thyme;
- 1 tsp baking soda;
- salt to taste.

You will need a muffin pan and muffin liners

How to prepare:

Preheat oven to 350° F. Melt the ghee in a mixing bowl. Add the almond flour and baking soda. Add eggs. Add the lemon thyme (use other herbs if you like) and the salt. Mix everything well. Add the bacon bits. Line a muffin pan with muffin liners. Pour the mixture into the muffin pan (to around ¾ full). Bake

for 18-20 minutes. Stick a toothpick the middle.
When it comes out clean, muffins are ready.

Preparation time: 15 minutes

Cooking time: 20 minutes

Total time: 35 minutes

Serving size: about 6 muffins, depending on the size of your muffin pan

Nutrition Information:

Calories: 300 | Fat: 28g | Carbohydrates: 7g | Sugar: 2g | Fiber: 3g | Protein: 11g

Cheese omelet with bacon

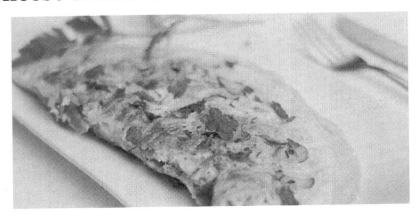

Ingredients:

- 3 eggs;
- 4-5 slices bacon;
- 1 Tbs of ghee or butter;
- a pinch of salt;
- a pinch of chili pepper.

How to prepare:

Cut the bacon strips into pieces and fry them over the high heat. Whisk eggs with salt and pepper in a bowl. Pour the mixture into a frying pan with the bacon, cover with a lid, and fry over low heat for about 10 minutes. Check occasionally for doneness.

Preparation time: 10 minutes
Cooking time: 10 minutes
Total time: 20 minutes
Serving size: 1 plate
Calories: 420 | Protein: 24g | Fat: 35g | Carbohydrates: 2g | Sugar: 1g

Fried eggs with cheese and nuts

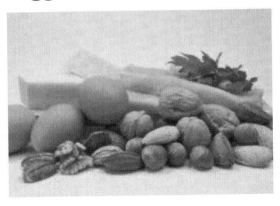

Ingredients:

- 2-3 eggs;
- 1 Tbs of olive oil;
- 1 oz cheese;
- 4 slices of bacon or ham;
- nuts (whichever you prefer);
- salt, pepper, herbs to taste.

How to prepare:

Fry the eggs in oil. Shred cheese, and put it on the eggs. Serve with nuts and other spices you may like.

Preparation time: 5 minutes
Cooking time: 10 minutes
Total time: 15 minutes
Nutrition information:
Calories: 236 | Fat: 19g | Carbohydrates: 0g | Fiber: 1g | Protein: 13g

Protein pancakes with cottage cheese

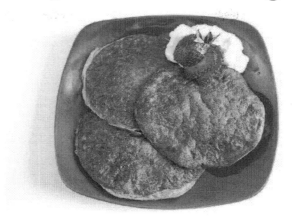

Ingredients:

- 2 oz cottage cheese;
- 2 egg whites;
- 1 tsp olive or coconut oil;
- a pinch of salt

How to prepare:

Separate egg whites and whip them with a fork. Heat a frying pan, grease it with oil, and pour in the beaten whites. When cooked on one side,carefully turn the whites to the other side. Mix cottage cheese with chopped herbs of your choice. Place the pancakes on a plate, top with the cheese mixture, and create whatever shape you like – an envelope, or roll , or eat it like a pancake.

Serving size: 1 plate. Calories: 139 | Protein: 13g | Fat: 9g | Carbohydrates: 1g |

Snacks

Spicy egg sandwich

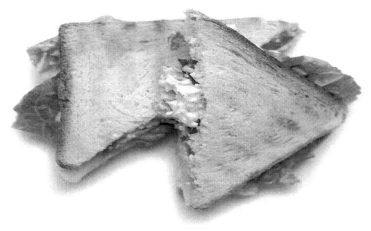

Ingredients:

- 2 eggs, hard boiled, diced;
- 2 Tbs of Greek yogurt;
- ½ tsp chili sauce;
- ½ bell pepper, diced;
- 2 tsp chopped of shallots;
- 2 slcies of whole grain bread;
- salt.

How to prepare:

Combine yogurt and chili sauce. Mix all the ingredients. Toast the bread. Place the eggs & vegetable mixture between slices of bread.

Calories: 290 | Carbohydrates: 22g | Proteins:10g

Chicken burrito

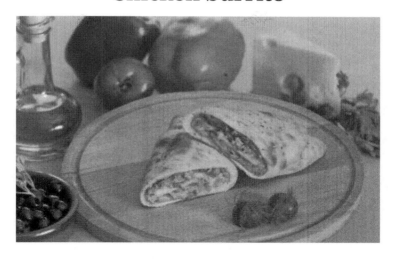

Ingredients:

- 1/2 lb chicken, minced;
- 2 tomatoes;
- 2 onions;
- 1 bell pepper;
- 1 Tbs olive oil;
- 1 Tbs mustard;
- 1/2 oz parsley, shredded;
- 1/2 oz dill, shredded;
- a pinch of black pepper;
- 2 slices pita bread.

How to prepare:

Heat the oil over medium heat for 1-2 minutes. Put the minced chicken into the frying pan. Add salt and pepper. Fry, stirring, for about 5-7 minutes. Put the chopped onion into warmed butter. Sauté until the onion is softened. Reduce heat and add the chopped bell peppers and tomatoes to the frying pan. Sauté for 10 minutes. Add the shredded parsley, dill, the ground black pepper and the mustard to the prepared minced chicken. Stir and warm for 2-3 minutes. Stiff the pita with the minced chicken and vegetables. Roll it. Do the same with the other pita bread.

Serving size: 2 rolls.

Nutrition information:

Calories: 260 | Carbohydrates: 16g | Proteins: 10g | Fat: 6g

Stuffed eggs

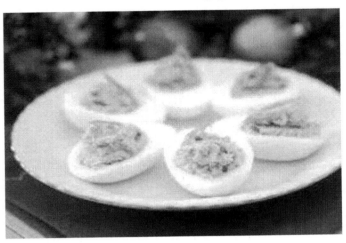

Ingredients:

- 3 eggs, hard boiled;
- 1 Tbs celery, diced;
- 1 stalk of green onion;
- 1 oz ham;
- 1 Tbs mayonnaise
- 1 tsp mustard;
- salt, pepper to taste.

How to prepare:

Cut the eggs in half. Remove yolks and mash them in a bowl. Put the egg whites aside, Chop the green onion and ham. Add to the mashed yolks. Mix with all the other ingredients and stuff the egg whites. Decorate with herbs.

Nutrition information:

Calories: 234 | Fat: 19g | Carbohydrates: 1g | Protein: 13g

Broccoli with Tofu

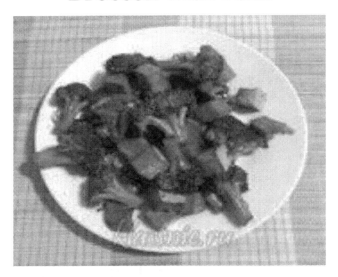

Ingredients:

- 3-4 oz tofu, cut in pieces;
- ½ of red onion, sliced;
- 10 broccoli florets;
- 1 clove of garlic;
- 1 inch of fresh ginger root;
- 4 Tbs sesame, coconut, or peanut oil (choose which you like);
- 2 Tbs soy sauce.

How to prepare:

Cook tofu pieces in oil in a frying pan on high heat until they are browned, stirring constantly. It will take a couple of minutes. Put aside. Fry broccoli, ginger, garlic and sliced onion, stirring well. Add soy sauce. Mix all cooked ingredients and heat them up for a minute. Serve, and enjoy it!

Serving size: 1 plate

Calories: 70 | Fat: 3g | Protein: 3g | Carbohydrates: 7g

Pepper stuffed with cottage cheese

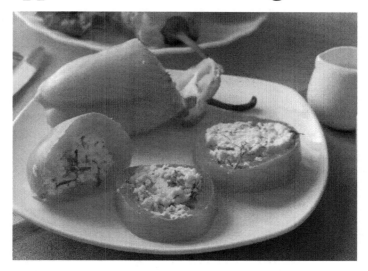

Ingredients:

- 5 oz cottage cheese;
- 1 clove of garlic, chopped;
- 2 Tbs parsley, dill, or fresh coriander;
- 4-5 green olives;
- 1 bell pepper.

How to prepare:

Finely chop garlic, herbs, and olives. Add cottage cheese and mix well. Stuff the bell pepper with the Mixture. For serving, slice the pepper and arrange the slices on a plage..

Preparation time: 5-7 minutes
Cooking time: 5 minutes
Total time: 10 minutes
Nutrition information:
Calories: 83 | Fat: 5g | Carbohydrates: 3g | Protein: 7g

Meat rolls without cooking

Ingredients:

- 4 slices of ham;
- a vegetable of your choice;
- 2 Tbs soft cheese or mayonnaise;
  herbs.

How to make:

Take a slice of ham. Put some soft cheese or mayo on top. Put a strip of pepper, or cucumber, or another vegetable you've chosen on top. Roll it.

Nutrition information:

Calories: 225 | Fat: 21g | Carbohydrates: 2g | Protein: 6g

Soft Tacos with Chicken and Avocado

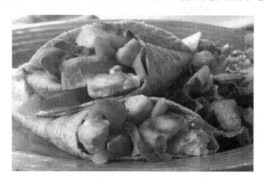

Ingredients:

- 1 tomato;
- 1 red onion;
- 1 avocado;
- 8-10 oz chicken fillet;
- a pinch of chili powder;
- a pinch of dried ground garlic;
- 1 Tsp olive oil;
- 2 tortillas;
- 2 oz salsa sauce;
- 2 oz cheese (cheddar).

How to prepare:

Cut the filet into small cubes, season it with chili and garlic, and fry on medium heat until golden brown. Finely dice the avocado, tomato, and onion, and mix them together Put all the ingredients on the tortillas, add salsa and grated cheddar. Fold and serve immediately.

Nutrition information:
Calories: 140 | Fat: 10g | Carbohydrates: 3g | Protein: 10g

Taco with fried cod and salsa

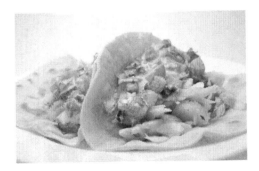

Ingredients:

- 2 tortillas;
- 7 oz cod fillets;
- 1 tomato;
- chili pepper to taste;
- 1 Tbs coriander leaves, chopped;
- 1 Tbs parsley, chopped;
- 1 oz red onion;
- 1 tsp lemon juice;
- salt to taste;
- 1 Tbs olive oil;
- 2 Tbs full-fat sour cream.

How to prepare:

Fry the cod in the oil. To make the salsa sauce:. chop the tomato and red onion. Finely chop herbs. Add pressed garlic. Dress with lemon juice and sour cream. Add salt and chili pepper. Mix the salsa well together. For serving, place cod on each tortilla and fold. Pour salsa on the top.

Nutrition information:
Calories: 125 | Fat: 9g | Carbohydrates: 3g | Protein: 6g

Lunch

Tamari marinated steak salad

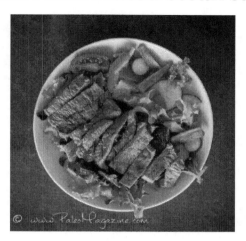

Ingredients:

- 2 large bunches (about 3 oz) of salad greens;
- 8-9 oz steak;
- ½ red bell pepper, sliced;
- 6-8 sour grapes or cherry tomatoes, cut into halves;
- 4 radishes, sliced;
- 4 Tbs olive or avocado oil;
- ½ Tbs fresh lemon juice;
- 2 oz tamari soy sauce (gluten-free);
- salt.

How to cook prepare:

Marinate the steak in the tamari soy sauce. Make the salad: toss the bell pepper, tomatoes, radishes, and salad greens with the oil, salt, and lemon juice. Cook or grill the steak with oil to the doneness you like. Put the steak on a platter for 1 minute, then cut it crosswise into slices.

Preparation time: 15 minutes
Cooking time: 10-20 minutes
Total time: 25-35 minutes
Nutrition Information:
Calories: 500 | Fat: 37g | Carbohydrates: 4g | Sugar: 1g | Fiber: 2g | Protein: 33g

Bacon wrapped chicken with garlic

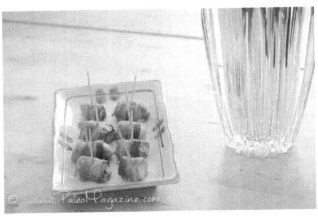

Ingredients:

- 1 chicken fillet, cut into small cubes;
- 8-9 thin slices of bacon, cut to fit the cubes;

- 6 cloves of garlic, minced.

How to prepare:

Pre-heat the oven to 400° F. Line a baking tray with aluminum foil. Add the minced garlic to a bowl and rub each piece of chicken with it. Wrap a bacon piece around each garlic chicken bite. Secure with a toothpick if necessary. Put the bacon wrapped chicken bites on the baking tray. Leave some space between them, so they're not touching. Bake until the bacon becomes crispy.

Preparation time: 15 minutes
Cooking time: 15-20 minutes
Total time: 35 minutes
Nutrition Information:
Calories: 260 | Fat: 19g | Carbohydrates: 5g | Sugar: 0 | Fiber: 1g | Protein: 22g

Easy zucchini beef sauté with garlic and coriander

Ingredients:

10 oz beef, sliced into 1-2 inch strips;
1 zucchini (about 10 oz), cut into one to two-inch-long strips;
¼ cup parsley or fresh coriander leaves, chopped;
3 cloves of garlic, diced or minced;
2 Tbs of tamari sauce;
4 Tbs avocado oil, coconut oil, olive oil (whatever you prefer).

How to prepare:

Put 2 Tbs of avocado oil (or other oil) in a frying pan on high heat. Place the strips of beef into the frying pan and brown them for a few minutes on high heat. When the meat is brown, add the zucchini strips and continue sautéing. When the zucchini is soft, add the tamari sauce, garlic, and parsley (or fresh coriander leaves). Let it stay for a few minutes more and serve immediately.

Serving size: about 10 oz.
Nutrition Information
Calories: 500 | Fat: 40g | Carbohydrates: 5g | Sugar: 2g | Fiber: 1g | Protein: 31g

Low-carb salad with liver and mushrooms

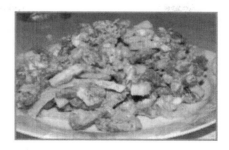

Ingredients:

- 3-4 oz beef liver;
- 1 egg, hard boiled;
- 1 oz dried mushrooms, reconstituted as directed on pakckage;
- 1 onion;
- 2 oz mayonnaise;
- 2 oz olive oil;
- salt, pepper to taste;
- dill for serving.

How to prepare:

Cut reconstituted mushrooms and liver into strips, add sliced egg. Place all the ingredients salad leaves. Sprinkle with dill.

Nutrition information:
Calories: 300 | Fat: 26g | Carbohydrates: 5g | Sugar: 2g | Fiber: 1g | Protein: 10g

Soups & Stews

Chicken Noodle Soup

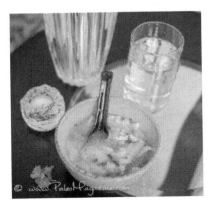

Ingredients:

3 cups chicken broth;
8-9 oz chicken breast, chopped into small bites;
2 Tbs of avocado oil;
1 stalk (2 oz) of celery, chopped;
1 green onion, chopped;
¼ cup fresh coriander leaves, finely chopped (approx 1/2 oz);

1 zucchini (approx. 3-4 oz) peeled
salt.

How to prepare:

Dice the chicken fillets. Add the avocado oil in a saucepan and sauté the chicken until it is well browned. Add chicken broth to the same pan and simmer. Chop the onions and celery, and add them to the saucepan. Chop the fresh coriander leaves, and put aside for the moment. Create zucchini noodles –

use a vegetable peeler to create long strands. Add zucchini noodles and fresh coriander to the pot. Simmer for a few minutes longer, add salt to taste, and serve immediately.

Serving size: 1 cup

Nutrition Information:
Calories: 300 | Fat: 17g | Carbohydrates: 6g | Sugar: 3g | Fiber: 2g | Protein: 34g

Broccoli & curry cream soup

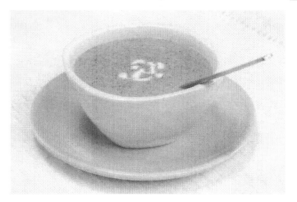

Ingredients:

- 6 oz broccoli, cut into pieces;
- 1¾ cups chicken broth;
- 1 oz cheese, grated;
- 3 oz cream;
- ½ oz ghee;
- 1 onion, sliced;
- 1 Tbs hot curry powder;

How to prepare:

Melt the ghee in a pot, put sliced onion in it. Fry the onion until it is brown. Pour the broth into the pot, and bring it to a boil. Add curry powder and stir. Put the broccoli into the broth and continue to simmer on medium heat for 10-15 minutes until the broccoli is soft. Use an immersion blender to blend cooked ingredients in the pot. To prevent lumps, gradually pour cream and cheese into the blended soup. Blend everything again.Serve the soup and enjoy!

Preparation time: 15 minutes
Cooking time: 20 minutes
Total time: 35 minutes
Serving size: 1 bowl
Calories: 300 | Protein: 11g | Fat: 36g |
Carbohydrates: 2g |

Soup with Poached Egg

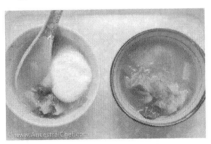

Ingredients:

- 2 eggs;
- 1 cup chicken broth;
- 1 small head of romaine lettuce, shredded;
- salt.

How to prepare:

Bring the chicken broth to a boil. Turn the heat to low and poach the 2 eggs in the broth for about 5 minutes. Remove the eggs and place each in a bowl. Add the shredded crunchy romaine lettuce to the broth and cook for a few minutes until slightly wilted. Pour the broth with the lettuce into the bowls.

Serving size: 1 bowl
Nutrition Information
Calories: 60 | Fat: 3g | Carbohydrates: 0g | Protein: 6g

Beef stew with mushrooms and vegetables

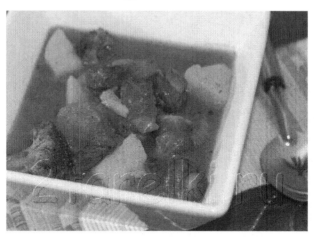

Ingredients:

- 8 oz beef meat (for stewing);
- 5 oz of champignons (or other mushrooms);
- 3 oz broccoli (fresh or frozen);

- 3 oz Brussels sprouts;
- 1 onion;
- 1 carrot;
- 1 stalk of celery;
- 1 Tbs of tomato paste;
- 2 Tbs of olive or coconut oil;
- salt and spices.

How to prepare:

Cut the beef into small pieces. Put some oil in a frying pan and fry the meat pieces until brown. Add some salt and spices. Cut mushrooms into quarters, and slice the carrot and onion. Use another pan for frying or grilling all the vegetables. Add more spices and salt, if desired. Put cooked meat and vegetables in a thick-bottomed pot. Let it stew for about 60 minutes on low heat.

Preparation time: 30 minutes
Cooking time: 60 minutes
Total time: about 90 minutes.
Nutrition Information
Calories: 180 | Fat: 11g | Carbohydrates: 0g | Protein: 18g

Mushroom cream soup

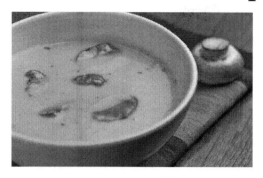

Ingredients:

- 1 tsp lemon juice;
- 1 small clove of garlic;
- 1 tsp olive oil;
- 2 Tbs ghee;
- 1 cup chicken broth;
- salt, black pepper to taste;
- 2 oz full-fat cream;
- 7 oz mushrooms.

How to prepare:

Wash mushrooms, set one aside for later and slice the rest.
Add the sliced mushrooms, garlic, ghee, oil and spices to a
saucepan, and sauté the mixture. . Add the broth and blend
the mixture with an immersion blender. Heat the soup,
adding the cream, gradually, to avoid lumps. Don't let it boil!
Pour into a bowl and decorate with the remaining sliced
mushroom.

Preparation time: 15 minutes
Cooking time: 20 minutes
Total time: 35 minutes
Serving size: 1 bowl
Nutrition Information
Calories: 115 | Fat: 11g | Carbohydrates: 0.5g | Protein: 2g

Cabbage & zucchini soup

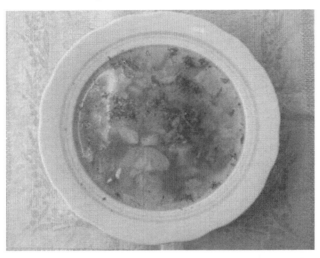

Ingredients:

- 7 oz cabbage;
- 3-4 oz zucchini;
- 3 oz carrot, sliced or cut into small cubes;
- 2 oz parsley root;
- 2 oz onion, sliced;
- 1 Tbs olive oil;
- 3 oz full-fat cream;
- 1¼ cups broth;
- salt, spices to taste.

How to prepare:

Boil the cabbage in the broth with the parsley root. Sauté the onion and carrot, and add them to the cabbage. After the vegetables are soft, add the cream. You can blend the soup or eat it as is.

Preparation time: 20 minutes
Cooking time: 25 minutes
Total time: 45 minutes
Serving size: 1 bowl
Nutrition Information
Calories: 30 | Fat: 2g | Carbohydrates: 1g | Protein: 2g

Chicken Soup with bacon and mushrooms

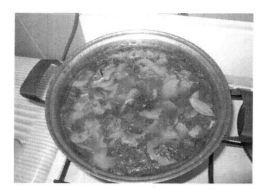

Ingredients:

- 2 cups chicken broth;
- 2 oz boiled chicken (from the broth);
- 2 oz bacon;
- 3 oz mushrooms;
- 1 onion;
- 1 carrot;
- 2 Tbs olive oil or ghee for cooking;
- 2 Tbs almond or sesame flour;
- salt, pepper.

How to prepare:

Finely cut mushrooms, onion, carrot, and bacon. Add the oil to a frying pan and fry the bacon, onion and carrot until soft. Put them into the boiling broth. Add flour, stirring thoroughly to prevent lumps. The flour makes the broth thicken. You can regulate the thickness of your soup by adding less or more flour. You can also add egg yolk to the soup if you like. Serve the soup with sour cream or ghee.

Stewed chicken livers

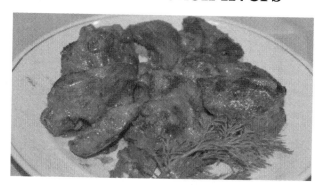

Ingredients:

- 10 oz chicken livers;
- 1 oz onion;
- 2 oz sour cream;
- 1 Tbs oil;
- salt.

How to prepare:

Slice onion and fry it in a pan with oil. Add livers and salt, and fry until the livers are half-cooked. Put in a pot, add sour cream, and stew for 20 minutes.
Serving size: one plate
Nutrition information:
Calories: 146 | Fat: 9g | Carbohydrates: 2g | Protein: 15g

Cream soup with shrimp

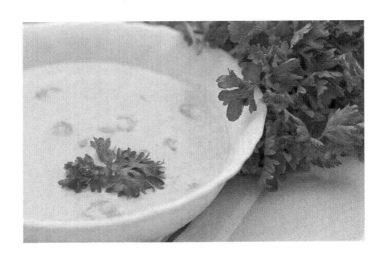

Ingredients:

- 2 oz shallot;
- 2 oz celery;
- 3 oz ghee;
- 2 cups broth;
- 2 oz clams with juice;
- 3 oz shrimp;
- 3 oz cod;
- 3 oz salmon;
- 2 cups of full-fat cream
- salt, pepper.

How to prepare:

Slice the onion and celery, and fry them until they are tender. Bring the broth to a boil, and add all the seafood. Decrease the heat. Add the remaining other ingredients, blend the soup, and bring back to a boil.

Nutrition information:

Calories: 16 | Fat: 1g | Carbohydrates: 0g | Protein: 2

Dinner

Cauliflower taboule salad

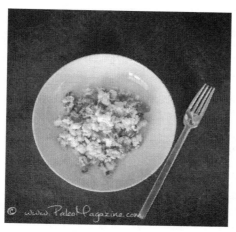

Ingredients:

- 3 oz cauliflower florets;
- 2 Tbs parsley;
- 6 mint leaves;
- 2 small tomatoes, diced;
- 2 cucumbers;
- 6 Tbs lemon juice;

- 2 Tbs of olive oil;
- Salt and pepper to taste;

How to preapre:

Make a couscous-like mass from the cauliflower florets by mincing them. Mix the cauliflower florets with finely cut herbs, tomatoes, lemon, olive oil, salt, and pepper. This tasty fresh salad may be used as a garnish or as the meal itself.

Nutrition Information:
Serving size: 1 plate
Calories: 80 | Fiber: 3g | Carbohydrates: 6g | Protein: 2g | Fat: 6g

Beef curry

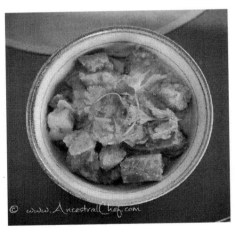

Ingredients:

- 1 lb beef, cut into cubes.
- 2 small onions, sliced;
- 1 Tbs curry powder;

- 1 tsp ground cumin (zira);
- 1 tsp ground coriander;
- 1 tsp turmeric powder;
- 1 tsp ground cardamon;
- ¾ cup of coconut milk;
- 2 carrots, sliced;
- 1 bell pepper, diced;
- 10 mushrooms, diced;
- 1 tsp freshly grated ginger;
- 2 cloves garlic, minced;
- ¼ cup fresh basil leaves, torn into pieces;
- salt;
- coconut oil for cooking.

How to prepare:

In a saucepan fry the beef and onions in the coconut oil for 5-6 minues on medium heat until the beef is browned, Add the spices, coconut milk, mushrooms, carrot, and bell peppers. Bring to a boil, Reduce heat, cover and simmer for 1 hour until the beef is done. You may need to add more liquid. Add the basil, garlic, ginger, and sal,t and simmer for 10 more minutes.

Nutrition Information:
Serving size: 1 bowl
Calories: 440 | Fat: 33g | Carbohydrates: 11g | Sugar: 2g | Fiber: 4g | Protein: 25g

Thai Chicken with cauliflower rice

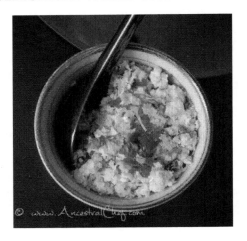

Ingredients:

- 1 head of cauliflower;
- 1 Tbs of ginger, freshly grated;
- 3 eggs;
- 3 chilies seeded and chopped (pick your favorite);
- 3 cloves of garlic, crushed;
- 3-4 cooked chicken breasts, shredded
- Salt;
- Coconut oil for cooking;
- 1 Tbs of tamari soy sauce;
- ½ cup of fresh coriander or parsley, chopped (for garnish)

How to preapre:

Break the cauliflower into florets and process in a blender until it forms a rice-like texture. Put the cauliflower into a large pan with the coconut oil and cook the cauliflower rice, stirring, on medium hear until it is soft. In a separate pan, scramble the eggs with some coconut oil. Add the scrambled eggs to the cauliflower rice. Add the ginger, garlic, and the chopped chilies. When the cauliflower rice mixture is soft, add the shredded chicken meat. Add the tamari soy sauce and salt to taste. Mix well. Garnish with fresh coriander or parsley.

Nutrition Information:
Serving size: 1 large bowl
Calories: 350 | Fat: 11g | Carbohydrates: 9g | Sugar: 4g | Fiber: 4g | Protein: 55g

Spinach salad with bacon and blue cheese

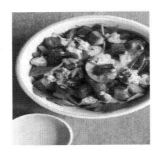

Ingredients:

- 2½ oz fresh spinach;
- 1 red onion, sliced;
- 3-4 Tbs blue cheese, crumbled;
- 2 oz almond nibs;
- 5 oz bacon strips.

How to prepare:

Fry the bacon strips on each side for 2-3 minutes. You don't need to add any oil because the bacon's fat is enough. Cut the bacon. For serving you need a salad plate. Place the spinach leaves on the bottom, then the sliced onion, cheese, and bacon. Top it up with the almond nibs. Use salad dressing if you like. This salad differs from the other green salads because of the blue cheese taste. It is an excellent low-carb salad.

Preparation time: 15minutes
Cooking time: 5-7minutes
Total time: 20 minutes
Serving size: 1 plate
Calories: 420 | Protein: 24g | Fat: 35g | Carbohydrates: 2g |

Grilled chicken skewers with garlic sauce

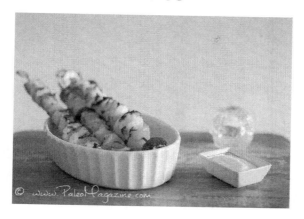

Ingredients:

- 8 oz chicken breast, cut into large cubes;
- 1-2 small onions, chopped;
- 2 bell peppers, chopped;
- 1 zucchini.

For the Garlic Sauce:

- 6-7 cloves of garlic;
- 1 tsp salt;
- about ¼ cup lemon juice;
- 1 cup olive oil.

Additional ingredients for the marinade:

- ½ cup olive oil;
- 1 tsp salt.

How to prepare:

Heat the grill to high. Soak wooden skewers in water first. For the garlic sauce, put the garlic cloves and salt into the blender. Then add ⅛ cup of the lemon juice and ½ cup of olive oil. Blend well for 5-10 seconds. It will change into the consistency of mayonnaise. Don't worry, if that does not happen – the sauce won't look amazing, but it'll still be tasty! Keep half the garlic sauce for serving. Take the other half of the garlic sauce and add the ½ cup of olive oil and salt. Mix well. Chop the onions, bell peppers, and zucchini into approximately 1-inch cubes or squares. Put them into the garlic marinade. Thread the vegetable and chicken cubes onto the soaked skewers and grill on high until the chicken cooked. Serve with the reserved garlic sauce.

Notes:

TIP: Making the mayo-like consistency can be a little bit difficult if you're new to it, so don't be upset if it looks a bit ugly. It still tastes good.

Nutrition Information
Serving size: 1 large plate
Calories: 580 | Fat: 33g | Carbohydrates: 11g | Sugar: 1g | Fiber: 3g | Protein: 55g

Pasta with chicken and basil

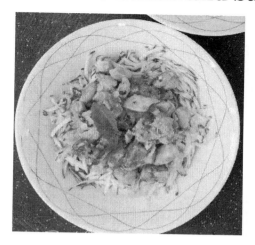

Ingredients:

- 2 chicken fillets, cubed;
- 2 Tbs ghee or coconut oil for cooking;
- 1 lb diced tomatoes;
- ½ cup basil, chopped;
- ¼ cup coconut milk;
- 1 clove of garlic, peeled, minced;
- salt;
- 1 zucchini, shredded.

How to prepare:

Sauté the cubed chicken in the ghee or coconut oil until done. Add tomatoes and salt. Simmer and reduce the liquid. Meanwhile, prepare the pasta. Shred zucchini in a food processor if you have one. Add the basil, garlic and coconut milk to the chicken and cook for a few minutes longer. Put half of the pasta into a bowl and top with the creamy tomato basil chicken.

Serving size: 1 large plate
Nutrition Information
Calories: 540 | Fat: 27g | Carbohydrates: 13g | Protein: 59g

Meat

Pork steak with parmesan

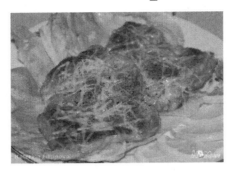

Ingredients:

- ½ lb pork steak;
- salt, black pepper;
- 1 oz Parmesan, grated;
- 1 Tbs lemon juice;
- 2 Tbs olive oil for cooking.

How to prepare:

Purchase an excellent cut of pork. Beat it a little with a kitchen mallet or with the dull side of a knife to tenderize and flatten it a little, Add salt and pepper. Let it rest for a few minutes. Fry it in a frying pan greased with the oil on very high heat for about 7-8 minutes on each side. Place the cooked steak on a plate, drizzle it with the lemon juice and cover with the grated Parmesan.

Serving size: one steak

Nutrition Information

Calories: 315 | Fat: 27g | Carbohydrates: 0 | Protein: 16g

Meat rolls

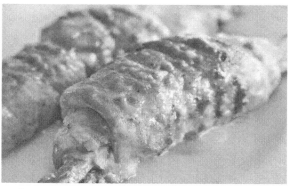

Ingredients:

- 5 oz pork or other meat;
- 2 oz cheese, sliced;
- 1 Tbs mayonnaise;
- 1 Tbs olive oil;
- salt, black pepper.

How to prepare:

Slice the meat. Beat the slices with a kitchen hammer.
Add salt and pepper. Let it rest for 10-15 minutes.
Place one cheese slice, on each slice of the meat. Roll
the cheese and meat. You can use kitchen twine to
prevent unrolling. Mix mayo and oil, and grease the
rolls with it. Preheat a frying pan, and add the rolls.
Fry over medium heat, turning on each side to brown
evenly. Before serving, take off the twine and season
with herbs. You can roll whatever stuffing you like
with the mea: asparagus, fried zucchini etc.
Serving size: 1 large plate

Nutrition information:

Calories: 340 | Fat: 28g | Carbohydrates: 0g |
Protein: 15g

Pan-fried pork tenderloin

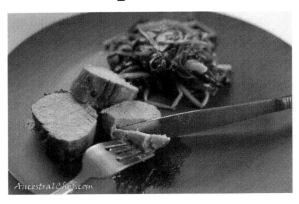

Ingredients:

- 1 lb pork tenderloin;
- salt and pepper to taste;
- 1 Tbs coconut oil

How to prepare:

Cut the pork tenderloin into equal halves. Put the coconut oil in a frying pan over medium heat. After the coconut oil melts, place both halves into the pan. Let the pork cook on one side. Once that side is cooked, turn to the other side. Keep turning and cooking until the pork is done to your taste. The pork will continue cooking for a while after you take it off the heat. Let the pork sit for a few minutes and then slice it.

Serving Size: 1 large plate

Nutrition Information:
Calories: 330 | Fat: 15g | Carbohydrates: 0 | Protein: 47g

Chicken with pesto and cream cheese

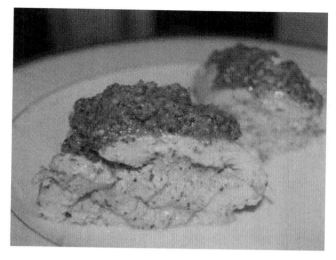

Ingredients:

- 1¼ lb chicken fillets;
- 2 Tbs ricotta;
- 1 tsp olive oil;
- salt, pepper to taste;

For pesto:
- 2/3 cup basil, fresh;
- 2 Tbs of walnuts;
- 1 clove of garlic;
- 2 Tbs Parmesan;
- ¼ cup of olive oil;
- salt.

How to prepare:

Roast the nuts in a frying pan over medium heat, stirring constantly until golden brown (2-3 minutes). Put all the ingredients for the pesto except the olive oil in a food processor, and make a purée. Add olive oil and mix well. Mix in ricotta. Slice the fillets, add salt and pepper, and beat them with a kitchen mallet to make thin fillets. Place a portion of the pesto filling on each fillet and wrap them. Grease a baking tray. Preheat the oven to 400° F. Put the fillets in the o ven for about 20 minutes.
Serving size: 1 large plate

Nutrition information:
Calories: 196 | Fat: 12g | Carbohydrates: 0 | Protein:

Fish & Seafood

Baked salmon with orange juice

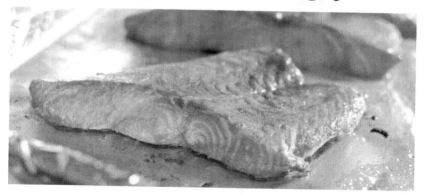

Ingredients:

- ½ **lb** salmon steak;
- juice of 1 orange;
- pinches of ginger powder, black pepper, and salt;
- juice of ½ lemon;
- 1 oz coconut milk;

How to prepare:

Rub the salmon steak with the spices and let it sit for about 15 minutes. Squeeze the orange into a bowl, with some pulp, and mix with the lemon juice. Pour the milk into the mixture. Put aluminum foil on a baking dish. Place the steak on it. Pour some sauce over the steak. Cover it with anoather sheet of foil. Bake at 350° F for 10 minutes.

Serving size: 1 portion

Calories: 300 | Protein: 7g | Fat 3g | Carbohydrates: 1g

Fried cod

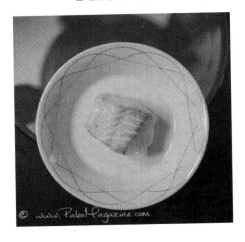

Ingredients:

- 4 cod fillets;
- 3 tsp of ghee;
- 6 cloves of garlic, minced;
- 1 Tbs garlic powder;
- Salt, spices.

How to prepare:

Melt the ghee in a frying pan. Add half of the minced garlic to the pan. Place the cod fillets in the pan and cook on medium to high heat. Add salt and garlic powder. As the fish cooks, it'll turn white. Wait for the white color to appear on the side of the fish and then flip the fish over. Add the rest of the minced garlic. Cook until the whole fillet turns a solid white color (it also flakes easily). Serve with the garlic and ghee which is left in the pan.

Serving size: 1 portion

Nutrition Information:
Calories: 160 | Fat: 7g | Carbohydrates: 1g | Protein: 21g

Tuna salad

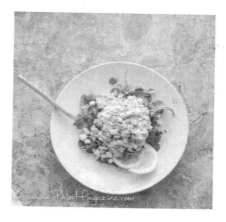

Ingredients:

- ⅓ cucumber,peeled and diced small;
- ½ avocado, diced small;
- 1 tsp lemon juice;
- 1 can (5-6 oz) of tuna;
- 1 Tbs of mayonnaise;
- 1 Tbs of mustard;
- salt, black pepper;
- salad greens.

How to prepare:

Mix the diced cucumber and avocado with the lemon juice. Flake the tuna and mix well with the mayo and mustard. Add the tuna mix to the cucumber and avocado. Add salt to taste. Prepare the salad greens: add olive oil and lemon juice to taste and toss well. Put the tuna salad on top of the salad greens. Add black pepper to taste.

One serving

Nutrition Information:
Calories: 480 | Fat: 40g | Carbohydrates: 13g | Sugar: 2g | Fiber: 8g | Protein: 40g

Mustard sardine salad

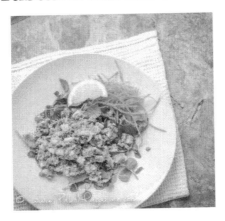

Ingredients:

- 1 can sardines in oil;
- ¼ cucumber, peeled and diced small;
- 1 Tbs lemon juice;
- ½ Tbs mustard;
- Salt and pepper to taste.

How to prepare:

Drain the oil from the sardines. Mash the sardines by using a fork. Mix well altogether: the sardines, diced cucumbers, lemon juice, and mustard. Add salt and pepper.

Serving: one salad

Preparation time: 15 minutes

Cooking time: 20 minutes

Total time: 35 minutes

Nutrition Information:

Calories: 250 | Fat: 19g | Carbohydrates: 0g | Protein: 25g

Baked shrimp with milk sauce

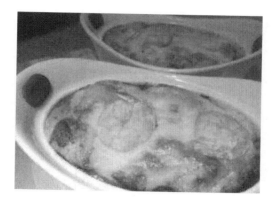

Ingredients:

- 6-7 oz shrimp;
- 1 oz of mozzarella;
- 4 oz milk sauce;
- 1 Tbs ghee.

How to prepare:

Cut boiled shrimps, put them into a baking dish. Pour milk sauce on them. Bake for 5-7 minutes in the oven.

Nutrition information:

Calories: 150 | Fat: 10g | Carbohydrates: 2g | Protein: 14g

Baked tilapia fillet

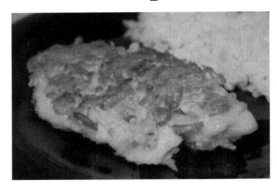

Ingredients:

- ½ lb tilapia or any white fish;
- 1 Tbs. ghee;
- 1 oz grated cheese;
- 1 Tbs. of mayonnaise;
- 1 small onion;
- ¼ tsp. dried basil;
- 1 Tbs lemon juice;
- Salt and pepper.

How to prepare:

Mix all ingredients, except fish. Cover a baking dish with aluminum foil, and bake tilapia for 4 minutes. Flip it, and bake 4 minutes more. Remove from the oven and pour sauce over it. Put it in the oven again, and bake for 3-5 minutes or until the sauce is brown and bubbly.

One serving

Nutrition information:

Calories: 570 | Fat: 60g | Carbohydrates: 1g | Protein: 15g

Veggies

Broccoli Salad

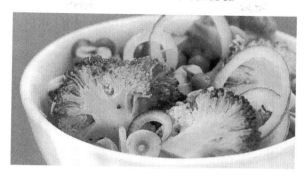

Ingredients:

- 10 broccoli florets (fresh or frozen);
- 2 red onions, sliced;
- 1 oz bacon, chopped into small pieces;
- 1 cup coconut cream;
- 1 tsp sesame seeds;
- salt.

How to prepare:

First, cook the bacon until crisp, and then cook the onions in the fat which is left from the bacon. Boil the broccoli florets for a couple of minutes (or you can use them raw). Mix the bacon pieces, onions, and broccoli florets with the coconut cream and salt. Top with sesame seeds. .

Nutrition Information:
Serving size: 1 portion
Calories: 280 | Fat: 26g | Carbohydrates: 8g | Sugar: 2g |Fiber: 3g | Protein: 10g

Spinach stir-fry

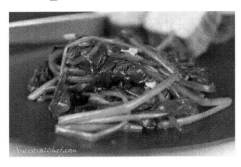

Ingredients:

- ¾ lb spinach;
- 3 Tbs almonds;
- Salt to taste;
- 1 Tbs coconut oil for cooking

How to prepare:

Put the oil into a large pot on high heat. Add the spinach and let it cook, stirring frequently. Once the spinach is cooked down and tender, add the salt and stir. Before serving, add almonds.

Preparation time: 5 minutes
Cooking time: 10 minutes
Total time: 15 minutes
Serving size: 1 portion
Nutrition Information:
Calories: 150 | Fat: 12g | Carbohydrates: 10g | Sugar: 1g | Fiber: 6g | Protein: 8g

Stuffed zucchini

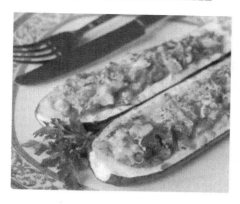

Ingredients:

- 2 zucchinis;
- 3 oz minced (whatever you like);
- salt, pepper, herbs, cheese to taste

How to prepare:

Cut zucchinis in half lengthwise. Scrape out the pulp and chop it finely. Mix it with the minced herb you've chosen, add salt, pepper, and stuff the mix back into the zucchinis. Preheat the oven to 350° F. Bake them until they're soft. Remove them and season with the cut herbs and grated cheese.
One serving
Nutrition Information:
Calories: 34 | Fat: 1g | Carbohydrates: 4g | Protein: 1g

Mushroom casserole

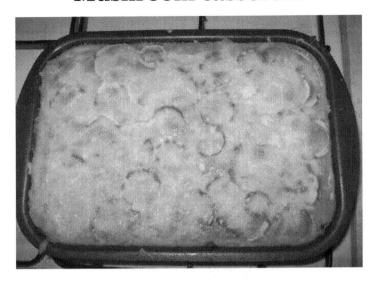

Ingredients:

- ½ lb mushrooms;
- 2 eggs;
- 1 oz of olive oil;
- 2 Tbs herbs;
- salt, pepper

How to prepare:

Boil washed mushrooms in salted water for 5-7 minutes until they are tender, Drain them. Whip eggs in a bowl, adding spices. Chop the mushrooms, add herbs, and put them in a greased baking dish. Pour the eggs into the dish with the mushrooms . The mushrooms should be covered with the eggs. Preheat the oven to 400° F, and place the baking dish inside.

Bake until it is slightly brown. Cooking time depends on how deep the dish is, on average, 20 minutes.
One serving
Nutrition Information:
Calories: 125 | Fat: 11g | Carbohydrates: 1g | Protein: 6g

Eggplant rolls:

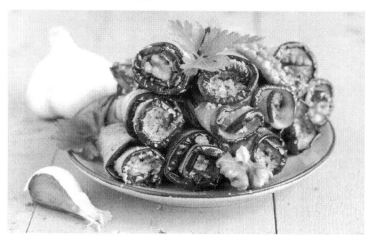

Ingredients:

- 2 eggplants;
- 3 Tbs olive oil for cooking;
- 2 oz full-fat cream cheese (or mayonnaise);
- 4 cloves garlic;
- 3 large sprigs of fresh dill;
- 3 green onions;
- 1 oz tomato;
- salt.

How to prepare:

Slice eggplants, salt the slices and set aside for 10 minutes. Mix chopped (or pressed) garlic with cheese and finely cut herbs. Fry eggplant slices in olive oil until they brown. Slice tomato and onion. Spread the cheese & garlic mix on each eggplant slice and top with a slice of tomato and onion. Roll each slice.
Servings: 2 portion

Nutrition Information:

Calories: 150 | Fat: 12g | Carbohydrates: 10g | Protein: 8g

Desserts

Keto mascarpone

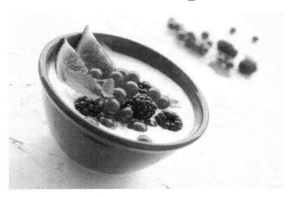

Ingredients:

- ¼ lb Mascarpone;
- 1 oz full-fat cream;
- 3-4 oz berries of your choice.
- 1-2 leaves of mint for decoration.

How to prepare:

Mix all the ingredients. Serve in a bowl and decorate with mint leaves.

Preparation time: 5 minutes
Cooking time: 5 minutes
Total time: 10 minutes
Serving size: 1 bowl
Nutrition Information:
Calories: 160 | Fat: 16g | Carbohydrates: 4g | Sugar: 1g | Fiber: 2g | Protein: 2g

Lemon cheesecake

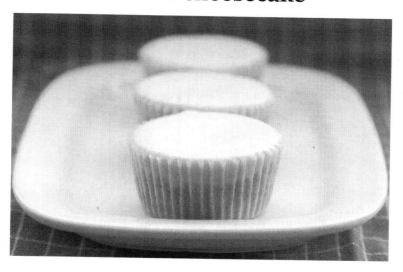

Ingredients:

- 6-7 oz of cream cheese;
- 2 oz full-fat cream;
- 1 Tbs lemon juice;
- a few drops of vanilla extract;
- peel of ½ lemon grated;
- Stevia.

How to prepare:

Take a large cup. Put cream and cream cheese in it. Mix them to a pudding-like consistency. Add the rest ingredients and mix again.

The secret of this cheesecake is that it doesn't need to be baked! It is a cold dessert. If your mouth is watering because of the masterpiece you've made, you can eat the dessert immediately after preparing, but it would be tastier if it is put for an hour or more in a refrigerator to let it solidify.

Preparation time: 5 minutes
Cooking time: 5 minutes
Total time: 10 minutes
Serving size: 1 portion
Calories: 220 | Protein: 6g | Fat: 17g | Carbohydrates: 2g | Sugar: 2g

Low-carb Cheesecake

Ingredients:

- 10 oz cream cheese;
- 2 eggs;
- 1 tsp vanilla extract;
- 1 tsp lemon juice;
- Stevia;
- 2 oz sour cream;

For the dough:
- 3 oz almond flour;

- 2 Tbs ghee;
- 2 Tbs low-carb jam (whatever taste you like).

How to prepare:

Mix all the ingredients for the dough, and place the dough into a deep baking form. Preheat the oven to the 375° F. Bake 8-10 minutes until it smells nice and gets brown. Meanwhile, prepare the filling by whisking the cream cheese until it is nice and fluffy. Gradually add the rest of the ingredients and keep on whisking for about a minute. Raise the oven heat to the 400° F. Pour the cheesecake filling on the already-baked dough in the baking form. Return it to the oven. Lower the heat to the 200°F. Bake for about 60 minutes, checking it from time to time. When the cake is firm, but still soft in the middle, the temperature should be about 155°F. Then take it out of the oven. Let it cool down. You can top it with strawberry jam or other sauce you like. You will be able to enjoy leftovers the next day with the fat coffee described in the next recipe.

Preparation time: 20 minutes
Cooking time: 90 minutes
Total time: 110 minutes
Serving size: 8 portions
Nutrition Information:
Calories: 240 | Fat: 28g | Carbohydrates: 2g | Sugar: 3g | Fiber: 3g | Protein: 6g

Fat Coffee

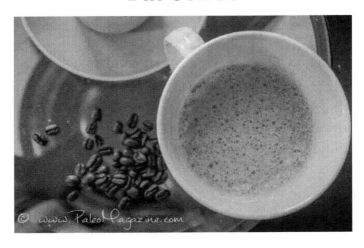

Ingredients:

- ½ Tbs ghee;
- ½ Tbs of coconut oil;
- 1 cup of your favorite coffee(or black tea)
- 1 Tbs almond or coconut milk.
- Stevia

How to prepare:

With a blender of shaker, mix the coffee, ghee, coconut oil, and Stevia or other zero-calorie sweetener and any flavoring you may like. This coffee boosts energy and keeps you from felling hungry. It is fantastic.

Nutrition Information:
Calories: 150 | Fat: 15g | Carbohydrates: 0g | Sugar: 0| Fiber: 0g | Protein: 0g

Keto lemon & coconut pancakes

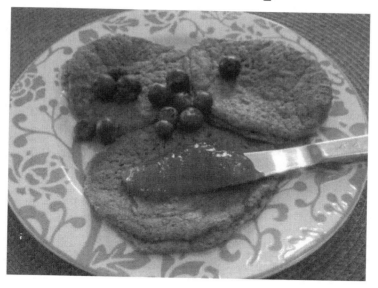

Ingredients:

- 1½ cups coconut milk;
- 4 eggs;
- 1 lemon;
- 4 Tbs chia seeds;
- 2 oz coconut nibs;
- 1 Tbs almonds, grated;
- 1 tsp baking soda;
- A few drops of vanilla extract;
- 2 Tbs coconut oil or ghee for cooking.

How to prepare:

Blend together all the liquid ingredients. Add the remaining ingredients except the oil or ghee and blend briefly forming the batter. Preheat a frying pan. Add some oil or ghee. Pour the batter into the pan using a tablespoon to form ovals. Fry on one side and flip over. Try not to overcook them.

Preparation time: 10 minutes
Cooking time: 20 minutes
Total time: 30 minutes
Serving size: 8 pancakes
Nutrition Information:
Calories: 300 | Fat: 28g | Carbohydrates: 7g | Sugar: 2g | Fiber: 3g | Protein: 11g

Cold melon & strawberry keto soup

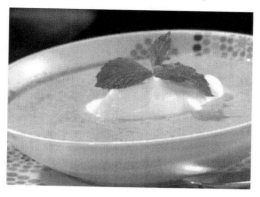

Ingredients:

- 1 cup ripe melon, cut into small pieces;
- 1 cup strawberries;
- ½ cup fresh green tea, prepared;
- 1 Tbs full-fat sour cream;
- 3-4 mint leaves for decoration.

How to prepare:

Blend melon and strawberries to purée-like consistency. Add tea and blend again. If you don't like strawberry seeds, peel the berries before blending. Pour into a bowl and decorate with mint leaves and sour cream

Preparation time: 10 minutes
Cooking time: 5 minutes
Total time: 15 minutes
Serving size: 1 bowl.

Protein berry cocktail

Ingredients:

- 3 oz coconut milk;
- 3 oz berries, frozen;
- 2 Tbs flax seeds;
- ½ -1 cup water, depending on the preferred consistency;
- 2-3 mint leaves for decoration.

How to prepare:

Mix all the ingredients together. Pour into a glass and decorate with a berry and mint leaves.

Nutrition information:

In 1 portion: Calories: 66 | Carbohydrates: 3g | Protein: 2g | Fat 5g

Almond butter fudge

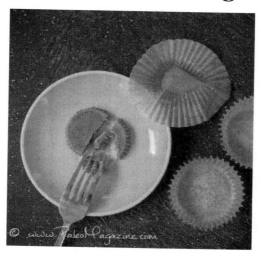

Ingredients:

- 1 cup of almond butter (unsweetened);
- 1 cup of coconut oil;
- ¼ cup coconut milk;
- 1 tsp vanilla;
- Stevia to taste.

How to prepare:

At first, melt the butter and oil together. Add all the other ingredients and blend well. Pour the mixture into a baking dish and leave it in the refrigerator for 2-3 hours for it to set. Cut into squares and serve.
Servings 2 portion
Nutrition information:
Calories: 650 | Carbohydrates: 0g | Protein: 2g | Fat 72g

Staples

Home-made mayo

Ingredients:

- 1 egg;
- 1 cup olive oil;
- 1 lemon (or 2 oz 3% vinegar);
- salt, mustard or garlic to taste

How to make:

In a bowl, mix the egg, salt and a teaspoon of oil. Use a fork to beat and homogenize the mixture. Gradually add the rest the of oil, continuously beating. At this point you can use a mixer. Add lemon juice or vinegar. Mix again. Add mustard or grated garlic or any other spices you like.
Carbohydrates per 3 oz – 2g

Egg sauce for the vegetables

Ingredients:

- 6-7 oz mayonnaise;
- 3 oz full-fat sour cream;
- 3 eggs;
- ¾ oz dill and/or parsley to taste.

How to prepare:

Hard boil the eggs. Remove yolks and mash them in a bowl, adding the mayo and sour cream. Mix it well. Add finely chopped herbs and mix everything well together.

Nutrition information:

Carbohydrates in every 3 oz – 2g

Guacamole

Ingredients:

- 2 big avocados;
- 3 Tbs onion, finely chopped;
- 2 Tbs cilantro, minced;
- 1 Tbs lemon juice;
- 1 chili pepper or jalapeño without seeds, chopped;
- 1 tomato, diced;
- ½ tsp salt;
- ¼ tsp ground black pepper.

How to prepare:

Cut avocados into halves, remove the pits and scrape the flesh into a bowl. Add other ingredients, and make a purée.

Nutrition information:

Carbohydrates in 8 oz – 6g, fiber – 4g

Garlic & nut sauce

Ingredients:

- 6 cloves garlic;
- 2 oz walnuts;
- 2 oz olive oil;
- 1/3 oz vinegar;
- herbs to taste.

How to prepare:

Mince the garlic. Mince the herbs. Grind the walnuts. Mix all the ingredinets together. The sauce is ready. Carbohydrates in every 3 oz– 3.75g

White Tartar sauce

Ingredients:

- 2 oz mayonnaise;
- 2 oz sour cream;
- 2 pickled cucumbers;
- salt

How to prepare:

Mix sour cream and mayo. Blend pickles or mince them finely. Add salt, and mix everything well.
You can also substitute pickled cucumbers with fresh ones.

Nutrition information:
Calories: 191 | Carbohydrates: 3g | Protein: 2g | Fat 19g

Peanut paste without sugar

Ingredients:

- 6-7 oz peanuts;
- 1 oz olive oil;
- ¼ tsp salt;
- ¼ tsp Stevia

How to prepare:

Blend peanuts into a sand-like mass. Add oil, salt, and Stevia, and mix well. Store it in glass jar.
Serving size: 4 portions
Nutrition information:
Calories in 3 oz: 592 | Carbohydrates: 8g | Protein: 23g | Fat 52g

Low-carb salad dressing

Ingredients:

- 1 Tbs apple vinegar;
- ½ Tbs basil infused vinegar;
- 2 tsp olive oil;
- Sweetener (such as Stevia) to taste.

How to prepare:

Mix vinegars and sweetener. Add oil. Blend well together. The dressing is ready.

30-day meal plan

Day 1

Breakfast: omelet with herbs

Lunch: meat steak with vegetables

Snack: stuffed pepper with cottage cheese

Dinner: pasta with chicken and basil

Day 2

Breakfast: cottage cheese, eggs, dried whole grain toast

Lunch: soup with cabbage and zucchini

Snack: keto mascarpone

Dinner: baked salmon with orange juice

Day 3

Breakfast: omelet, tomato, basil, sheep's milk cheese

Lunch: almond butter fudge

Snack: broccoli salad

Dinner: white fish, egg with spinach, cooked in coconut oil.

Day 4

Breakfast: 3 scrambled eggs with spinach, cheese, sausages

Eggs are a healthy, nutrient-dense food. Increased cholesterol in your blood is not because of cholesterol in food, so, you can eat eggs for your pleasure — they are full of protein and lutein, and make you feel full for hours. Make a healthy omelet with some cheese, crumbled sausage, and shredded spinach which is packed with magnesium and potassium, too. Add some sea salt, and you'll have a big dose of electrolytes that are so vital to maintaining energy and reducing headaches.

Lunch: Spinach salad

Salads are your best friends when in ketosis because they provide lots of food to fill you up. A bunch of spinach with some red onion, bacon, a little tomato, and a hot sauce vinaigrette is quick and delicious.

Snack: Burger with cheese and guacamole.

Dinner: chicken soup with bacon and mushrooms

Day 5

Breakfast: fried eggs with bacon and mushrooms.

Lunch: salmon steak

Snack: nuts

Dinner: beef, buckwheat, tomato

Day 6
Breakfast: cheese and fat coffee

Lunch: stuffed zucchini

Snack 1: chicken burritos

Snack 2: pancakes

Dinner: steak with eggs and salad.

Day 7
Breakfast: bacon and eggs
The keto followers adore it. 2-3 fried eggs and some bacon might not sound like much, but it's full of protein that will mke you feel full of energy all morning.

Lunch: Boiled meat, vegetables

Snack: cold melon & strawberry keto soup

Dinner: Thai chicken with cauliflower rice

Day 8
Breakfast: avocado, baked eggs
Cut avocado in two, crack an egg into the seed hole and bake it until the egg sets.

Lunch: chicken and hummus lettuce wraps

It is a quick, healthy lunch that provides a protein punch and without a ton of calories.

Snack 1: meat rolls without cooking

Dinner: pan-fried pork tenderloin

Day 9

Breakfast: why not eat leftovers from the last dinner?

Lunch: low-carb cheesecake

Snack: soft tacos with chicken and avocado

Dinner: mushroom cream soup

Day 10

Breakfast: scrambled eggs, grilled sausages, tomatoes

Lunch: Tacos
Choose your favorite taco recipe. Take some beef, and use romaine leaves for shells. Add some full-fat sour cream and cheese, and you'll never miss the tortillas.

Snack: Keto soup

Dinner: baked trout

Day 11

Breakfast: fat coffee with lemon cheesecake

Lunch: Taco salad
Take your leftover tacos and make a taco salad. Top
with sour cream, and some grated cheese. Protein,
fat, and veggies will fill you up all day!

Snack: spinach salad with bacon and blue cheese

Dinner: Thai chicken with cauliflower rice

Day 12

Breakfast: spinach salad
Salads are your best friends when in ketosis because
they provide lots of food to fill you up. A bunch of
spinach with some red onion, bacon, a little tomato,
and a hot sauce vinaigrette is quick and delicious

Lunch: grilled chicken skewers with garlic sauce

Snack: stuffed eggs

Dinner: Pork and roasted veggies
A nice pork roast rubbed down with cumin, salt,
and garlic will give you leftovers for days and it is
pretty cheap. Add some Brussels sprouts, broccoli,
or cauliflower that have roasted in the oven until
brown and delicious, and you've got a real comfort
meal.

Day 13
Breakfast: bacon lemon thyme breakfast muffins

Lunch: broccoli salad

Snack: mustard sardine salad

Dinner: cabbage & zucchini Soup

Day 14
Breakfast: asparagus and egg

Lunch: bacon and eggs

Snack: cream soup with shrimp

Dinner: boiled turkey with white tartar sauce

Day 15
Breakfast: protein pancakes with cottage cheese

Lunch: Salad
Take 2-3 cups of lettuce, crumble some bacon and slice a medium tomato. Mix with 2-3 tablespoons of mayo and a splash of hot sauce. Delicious, filling, full of fiber and healthy fats! Easy! The mayo sounds weird as a dressing, but it is superb! Add some avocado chunks to boost potassium.

Snack: spicy egg sandwich

Dinner: Baked salmon with asparagus
You will appreciate the effortless cooking of salmon,
for sure! A simple sauce of butter, lemon juice,
chopped garlic, some salt, and pepper will enhance
the natural flavor of the salmon. Easy dinner (with
leftovers, if you plan ahead) that's full of nutrition,
protein, healthy fat, while keeping your carbs low.

Day 16
Breakfast: eggs with tomato

Lunch: cheesecake and coffee

Snack: ham and cheese with nuts

Dinner: beef stew with mushrooms and vegetables

Day 17
Breakfast: cheese omelet with bacon

Lunch: cottage cheese, walnuts, hot sauce

Snack: protein cocktail

Dinner: pork steak with parmesan

Day 18

Breakfast: 3 fried eggs, protein cocktail, 1 oz cheese

Lunch: bacon lemon thyme breakfast muffins

Snack: taco with fried cod and salsa

Dinner: lemon cheesecake

Day 19

Breakfast: omelet, ½ grapefruit, unsweetened tea

Lunch: easy zucchini beef sauté with garlic and coriander

Snack: broccoli with tofu

Dinner: soup with poached egg

Day 20

Breakfast: cheese omelet with bacon

Lunch: Tuna salad lettuce wraps
It is effortless and delicious, doubly so when you chop some fresh avocado with it.

Snack: spicy egg sandwich

Dinner: chicken soup with bacon and mushrooms

Day 21

Breakfast: stuffed eggs

Lunch: baked salmon with orange juice

Snack: dessert

Dinner: broccoli & curry cream soup

Day 22

Breakfast: boiled eggs, yogurt

Lunch: chicken soup, salad

Snack: meat rolls without cooking

Dinner: boiled chicken, veggies

Day 23

Breakfast: eggs with cheese and nuts

Lunch: pasta with chicken and basil

Snack: dessert

Dinner: Thai chicken with cauliflower rice

Day 24

Breakfast: protein pancake with cottage cheese

Lunch: stewed chicken liver

Snack: eggplant rolls

Dinner: grilled chicken skewers with garlic sauce

Day 25
Breakfast: cheese omelet with bacon

Lunch: baked salmon with orange juice

Snack: dessert

Dinner: mushroom casserole

Day 26
Breakfast: fat coffee, almond butter fudge

Lunch: easy zucchini beef sauté with garlic and coriander

Snack: lemon cheesecake

Dinner: tuna (canned), spinach salad

Day 27
Breakfast: eggs and bacon, fat coffee

Lunch: mushroom casserole

Snack: spinach stir-fry

Dinner: fried cod with garlic

Day 28

Breakfast: scrambled eggs with guacamole

Lunch: bacon wrapped chicken with garlic

Snack: baked tilapia fillet

Dinner: chicken with pesto and cream cheese

Day 29

Breakfast: cheese omelet with bacon

Lunch: cauliflower taboule salad

Snack: baked shrimp with milk sauce

Dinner: pasta with chicken and basil

Day 30

Breakfast: keto lemon and coconut pancakes

Lunch: chicken noodle soup

Snack: seafood & celery salad

Dinner: eggplant rolls

Conclusion

A ketogenic diet, or keto diet, is a very low-carb diet, which turns the body into a fat-burning machine. It has many potential benefits for weight loss, health, and performance, but also has some potential initial side effects. A keto diet is designed to result in ketosis. It is possible to measure and adapt to reach optimal ketone levels for health, weight loss, and for physical and mental performance.

You can use a ketogenic diet just to improve health and not necessarily to lose weight, of course.

Keto is a lifesaver for many people. It is nice to feel satisfied, to eat delicious food and still to lose weight. Keep in mind: the more physical training and activity you have, the faster fat burns.

Made in the USA
San Bernardino, CA
21 February 2019